More Praise for
The Power *of* Positive Choices

"You hold in your hands a small, potent, and magical book. Make a positive choice right now; read it. Absorb its wisdom. Act on the insights you gain and you're on your way to experiencing a renewed joy in living."

—LYNN A. ROBINSON, author of *Divine Intuition: Your Guide to Creating a Life You Love*

"The simple process of Addition and Subtraction makes it so easy to incorporate dynamic change in your life. *The Power of Positive Choices* will transform the way you care for yourself."

—DEBORAH KNOX, co-author of *Life Work Transitions.com: Putting Your Spirit Online*

"A gem of a book. This simple guide to life transformation provides the structure and support to find your true self."

—LUCIA CAPACCHIONE, PH.D., art therapist and author of *Visioning: Ten Steps to Designing the Life of Your Dreams*

"Gail has the ability to show us how to move our lives forward with power, dignity and grace.... She is truly the Goddess of Creativity!"

—LORETTA LAROCHE, author of *Relax—You May Have Only a Few Minutes Left*

"A highly sensible guide to help you stop daydreaming and start making the choices that are ultimately fulfilling."

—TALANE MIEDANER, author of *Coach Yourself to Success*

The
Power *of*
Positive
Choices

Adding and
Subtracting
Your Way
to a Great Life

Gail McMeekin, M.S.W.

Foreword by Barbara Sher

CONARI PRESS
Berkeley, California

This book is dedicated
to your divine capacities for creativity
and change, in harmony with
the higher good.

Conari Press books are distributed by Publishers Group West.

ISBN: 1-57324-573-9

Book and Cover Design: Suzanne Albertson
Author Photo: Gretje Ferguson

Library of Congress Cataloging-in-Publication Data

McMeekin, Gail E.
    The power of positive choices : adding and subtracting your way to a great life / Gail McMeekin.
        p.   cm.
    Includes bibliographical references.
    ISBN 1-57324-573-9
    1. Self-actualization (Psychology) 2. Choice (Psychology)
I. Title.

BF637.S4 M295 2001
158.1—dc21   00-013018

Printed in the United States of America on recycled paper.

01 02 03 04   DATA   10 9 8 7 6 5 4 3 2 1

The Power *of* Positive Choices

Preface

Do you long to feel the joy of living? Do you crave time for friends and family, new experiences, the luxury of your own creative thoughts? These are healthy wishes. By learning the art of Positive Choices, you can reprioritize your life and initiate many more memorable moments. We live in a frantic world—bombarded by more information than we can possibly assimilate, assaulted by media negativity, and exhausted from a lack of leisure. Gone are the days when we had time to sit still and connect with ourselves and our creative impulses— we're all on overdrive. To stay in touch with who you are at this moment in time, you must learn to filter out the things that compromise your serenity. By reading this book, you have chosen to dance with the magic of change. Congratulations. Hidden gains await you.

This is an intentionally small book, but it is potent. The Positive Choices technique is both simple and extremely powerful. Each chapter focuses on one of the letters in the words *Positive Choices*. Each letter reveals an axiom for you to ponder, and includes exercises called "Inquiries" to help you to take a series of growth-inducing actions. The letters in the words *Positive Choices* correlate with specific perceptions and action steps. Together they represent a holistic approach that integrates Doing with Being. Take your time with these concepts, divulge your truths, and engage with your innovation process. The stories of other men and women who have brought Positive Choices into their lives will light your way on this journey. Your life's path will unfold in its right time and in its unique form.

Foreword

by Barbara Sher, author of
It's Only Too Late If You Don't Start Now

These days, we have more opportunities and more resources than ever before, and still, even with all these benefits, we often have a half-conscious, nagging feeling that we've somehow lost our way. Being lost is not the worst thing in the world; after all, if you know you're lost, you can sit down and start thinking. Maybe you'll find a map or remember some instructions or figure out a way to read the terrain or send up a flare for help.

It's a bigger problem to be lost and not admit it. We may sense that something's not right, but we're too busy to think about it. Or the road looks so familiar, it's hard to believe we could be lost. You know what to do today because you did it yesterday and you'll do it again tomorrow. Granted, you always have more than you can do and a nagging "To Do" list, but if you keep at it, you might get it together one of these days.

We never stop to ask ourselves the simple, powerful

question Gail McMeekin asks us at the very beginning of this book: Is everything okay? We don't ask ourselves because we're not sure we want the answer. What if everything isn't okay? What are we supposed to do about it? Tear our lives apart and start over? If that's what we have to do, maybe it's better to not ask the question in the first place. But that's where this book shines. Maybe you don't control the universe, it tells us, but you do control your life choices. By making one small choice at a time, you can turn your life around.

Although we had met briefly a few years earlier, I came to know Gail McMeekin one day when we sat in her magical Victorian house in Boston while she interviewed me for her book, *The 12 Secrets of Highly Creative Women.* I believe I found out as much about Gail that day as she did about me. I already knew she had been a psychotherapist and a career and creativity coach for more than twenty-five years. But that day we spent together I learned how deeply she believes in the potential for people to change their lives—one step at a time. I discovered that her sense of timing is unique, and that she has a rare respect for the impact real life events can have on us. "Change has to be timed well," she said, "with a lot of respect for the unexpected challenges life can hand us."

I learned more about Gail as she took me through the house she and her husband had restored with love and care. The house is unforgettable. As soon as you see it from the street, you know it's lovable and honest. But the more you explore, the more you find: a perfect detail, an unexpected charming corner, quietness, affection, and humor at every step. No junk or clutter. What struck me as most typical of Gail herself were the many clever solutions to small, important needs: the need for a beam of sunlight on the stairs, for a cozy place to curl up and read where no one will find you, or for a white flower in a bud vase to light up a dark corner.

At the time, I didn't know about Gail's workshops. I've since learned that they're famous. They grew out of her early stress seminars when she realized that relaxation techniques weren't enough to melt stress—you had to resolve the problems that caused the stress in the first place. She's designed a system that takes on reality: if something's wrong, don't just breathe deeply. Face it. Then you can change it—element by element, one at a time, subtracting something that you know isn't right, adding something that feels very right. It's as simple as putting in a garden. And as powerful.

So open the pages and read this generous book. Let yourself slow down to the pace of the writing with Gail's wonderful sense of timing. Along with her words, the pace itself will help you see where you are, remind you where you want to be, and show you how to find your way.

Imagine taking an early morning walk to the top of a cliff. As you stand basking in the stillness and the majesty of the view, suddenly the cliff transforms into a tall narrow spire. You find yourself confined to a small circle of stone. Your path to the bottom has vanished. There is no turning back—only a future for you to create. In front of you appear two bridges leading into the mist. Inscribed on the entrance to the first bridge are the words, *The Same.* On the second bridge the inscription reads, *Positive Choices.*

Panic sets in. It looks like you have to select one bridge or the other to escape. You approach the first bridge again and ponder the inscription. *The Same? The same what?* You climb to the top of the steps, and suddenly, a small television monitor drops down from the archway. The screen reads, "If you choose this bridge, you will return to your life exactly as it was before you climbed this cliff." A video then begins to play scenes from a typical day in your life, over and over. Finally you yell, "Stop!" The screen darkens for a moment. But then it flashes on again with the words, *Stay Tuned.*

Shaken, with the chill of the mountain air invading your bones, you ponder the options. *My life isn't so bad,* you protest. *Sure, I'd love to have some new adventures, and there are circumstances that I'm unhappy about, but what do I expect? I think I'll just walk onto this bridge and go home. That's the sensible thing to do. Why is this happening to me anyway?*

You hear music and the next video begins. On the screen are a series of questions for you to answer. A voice instructs you to begin the Self-Test, responding to questions about your life with a Yes or No answer.

Self-Test on Life Fulfillment

1. Are you truly happy?

    ____Yes   ____No

2. Are you pleased with the person you are?

    ____Yes   ____No

3. Are you challenged and passionate about your personal and professional lives?

    ____Yes   ____No

4. Are you expressing yourself authentically in your relationships?

    ____Yes   ____No

5. Are you meeting the goals you have set for yourself?

    ____Yes   ____No

6. Are you content with the choices you have made in your life?

   ____Yes   ____No

7. Are you living the life of your dreams?

   ____Yes   ____No

8. Do you feel in control of your destiny?

   ____Yes   ____No

Score: Add up the number of Yeses and Noes

   ____Yeses   ____Noes

A voice booms over the monitor, "You must tell the truth or you will fail the test and have to complete it again." You reconsider a few answers and surrender to the fact that many of your answers are "Noes." You are not living the life you dreamed of, and you don't feel in charge. Your inner voice whispers, "If you have all of these negatives, maybe you should check out the message at the other bridge. Perhaps you are missing an opportunity to move beyond the ordinary to something extraordinary."

Reluctantly, you step toward the bridge labeled "Positive Choices." The mist parts slightly and reveals a small chest a few feet in front of you. This tiny treasure chest glistens with amethyst and tanzanite stones. You sit on the top stair, place the chest in your lap, and lift the lid in anticipation.

Inside you find a piece of purple notepaper and, next to it, a small book. The title of the small book reads *The*

Power of Positive Choices. You unfold the purple note, which reads as follows:

> It is no accident that you are here today. You know deep within that your life is at a choice point. Perhaps you know exactly what's next but can't make the first move. Or maybe you just know there's something missing. What if you had the power to re-create your life? What would you hang onto and what would you let go of? What are your dreams and wishes? Once you identify and subtract what's undermining the joy in your life and add in Positive Choices that express your uniqueness, a momentum begins. You do have the power to transform your life—at your own pace, in your own time. The simple art of making Positive Choices will help you, step by step, to manifest the vision of the life you want. Interested? Do you have the courage to take a risk and stake a claim on what you truly desire? If you choose this path, hold onto the treasure chest and walk across this bridge.

Acknowledging the restlessness and discontent you've concealed from yourself, you make a daring decision. Intrigued and ready for a life closer to your ideals, you salute your inner voice, daringly choose the bridge of Positive Choices, and march into the mist. Instantly, you float downward, landing next to your car in the moonlight, your hand clutching the treasure chest. You've just initiated a new chapter in your life. Unknown possibilities abound. Feeling excited, you drive home filled with a new sense of promise. Once inside your home, you curl up in your comfy chair, remove this book from your jeweled chest, and begin to read.

Keep track of your insights while you write in a lovely journal or on a notepad. You will find the journal especially useful for answering the questions and doing the exercises in the Inquiries that appear in each chapter of the book. Keeping the journal also lets you follow your progress as you gradually release the negative elements in your life and move more and more into Positive Choices.

part I

The
Power *of*
Positive

In the context of this book, the term *Positive* means becoming proactive so that you can increase your life's bounty of health and happiness. *Positive* implies being assertive and decisive. It is the opposite of being negative and passive. When you embark on a mission to re-create your life, your self-confidence ascends. You embrace the Positive and delete the negative. A life of Positive Choices is a vision of the life you long for. It is an affirmation and an intention that you are willing to change your beliefs and your behaviors to attain your goals.

By choosing the bridge of Positive Choices, you will leave many negative people in your wake. You will no longer want to play the game of who is suffering more — it will bore you. Instead, you will be intrigued by people who think Positively like you and who initiate changes in their lives that reflect that philosophy. Your Positive energy will exhilarate the receptive people around you and inspire them to follow their own excitements.

Chapter 1

P Is for
Priorities

Your choices determine the quality of your life experience. The act of making choices implies the chance or the power to select one option over another. Positive Choices are life choices elected to support your body, mind, and spirit. Negative life choices, such as doing unsatisfying work or staying in a destructive relationship, undermine your joy of living. They drain you of your precious life energy and potential. Yet, in the wake of stress and life adversities, we often forget that we *do* have the power to re-create our lives by Adding and Subtracting Positive and negative life choices. In fact, learning and then implementing this basic yet challenging technique empowers you to claim the life you truly desire.

Do we have total control over every life choice? No. Wanda would love to be tall and lithe and sing like Barbra Streisand. Again and again in her life she has found herself thinking, *If only I were 5 foot 8 inches tall and could sing....* But, instead, she's 5 foot 1 inch short and was shamed out of junior choir for singing off key. Is she totally helpless to her fate? No. She could wear shoes to make her look taller, and her musical friends insist that she could learn to sing if she practiced. But high heels kill her feet, and Columbia Records will probably never chase her down to cut a solo album no matter how much she practiced. So Wanda has decided to live with her limitations and forgo the uncomfortable shoes and voice lessons. She's chosen to leverage her natural talents and let go of her "if only" fantasies.

INQUIRY *Are there any "if only" life choices haunting you? If so, what are they? Are these life choices impossible or possible? If they are indeed possible life choices, are they important enough to you so that you can select one or more of them and dedicate your energy toward mastery of it? Make note of the life choices that you want to pursue and those you choose to release. As suggested in the Introduction, use your journal to answer the questions and do the exercises in these Inquiry sections.*

Gratitude for who you are and what you have already manifested in your life creates a strong foundation of support while you walk through the fires of change. Ponder all the "riches" currently present in your life—your abilities and interests, people you cherish, environments that nurture you, your health, Nature's glory, and any other manifestation you may want to acknowledge. The madness around us often eclipses our appreciation of walks on the beach, connections with people who nourish our souls, or exciting work. Resolve to thank the universe regularly for the gifts you already have.

INQUIRY *What are the good things in your life? Write down all of the life choices or gifts that you are grateful for and want to celebrate today. Again, use your journal to answer the questions and do the exercises in these Inquiry sections.*

Many people find the number of possible life choices overwhelming. There is a seemingly endless selection. You could be a gypsy and live in a foreign land, start a successful restaurant, or take in homeless children. Determining your priorities is an essential sorting-out process. Noting which life choices infuse your life with passion and fulfillment helps you to elevate these life choices to top priorities. What do you desire most?

Clearing out the things in your life that don't work opens up an entire range of new options and possibilities. The older I get the more I see the wisdom in the axiom, "Less is more." Take a mantle over a fireplace, for example. Mantles often hold family photographs, flowers, and candlesticks. Yet, I've been noticing lately how many people's mantles appear packed with too much *stuff*. Recently, I took everything off my mantle and realized that this myriad of objects was hiding the beautiful hand-carved woodwork. After pondering the image that I wanted to project, I selected a pair of thin but elegant candlesticks and a crystal clock to sit on the newly exposed shelf. These three pieces were my priorities to display. I wanted to study these three objects for a while and savor their combination. Formerly, these objects and the woodwork were buried in my maze of excess.

Simplification is a guiding principle for the Positive Choices part of the book. You can't do it all, have it all, or experience it all. So you must choose your priorities wisely and carefully. To do that, you must be willing to release the old, the excessive, and the outgrown in both the material and the psychological worlds.

INQUIRY *Given the limitations of time and energy, what principles, activities, or people do you choose to make the Focal Points or Top Priorities in your life? Make a list in your journal. If your list is longer than ten items, I suggest that you shorten it. Post your top priorities on a file card and review them daily to verify your selections. Freely edit until your list presents the real truth.*

Many people resist having a focus in their lives and jump from career to career, relationship to relationship, or project to project. This process of constant shifting can leave you feeling drained and frustrated. Does choosing a focus involve a loss? Of course. If you choose to write one book now and postpone another, or decide to live on the ocean rather than in the desert, you have selected one option at the expense of the other. But by focusing, you connect more powerfully with your opted choice. If you don't like it, you can change it. Or if you live on the ocean, you can vacation in the desert. Allow your top priorities to serve as a daily framework for your time.

Chapter 2

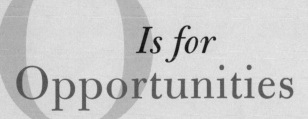

Is for
Opportunities

Selecting life priorities precipitates another rendezvous with the ever-challenging question, "Why are you here?" This Positive Choices chapter propels you toward claiming your personal mission and power. Openness to new opportunities engages your evolution process. Now that you have chosen your current Positive Choices—those priorities that form the foundation for your lifetime—you want to engage the Addition Factor.

First, let's check in with your inner voice to see if you have been getting any signals about what's missing from your life. Have you recently been aware of your inner messenger or intuition either whispering softly in your ear or screaming loudly to pay attention *now?* Exactly what is your inner voice telegraphing? Burnout, boredom, pain, death, job loss, or crisis can heat up the intensity of your messenger's voice. Have your been ignoring this inner guidance, or is your messenger currently silent? If you've been hiding from your messenger, it's time to end the game and listen. You may experiment with our cultural distractions—drugs, television, overwork, food, or gambling—but these distractions only delay your encounter with these internal clues. Eventually your inner voice will win out, and you will be forced to consider what's being said. By listening now, you may prevent a later negative crisis, like an illness or an accident, that will shock you into tuning into yourself. Trust that your inner messenger is working on your behalf.

INQUIRY *Does your messenger have a message for you and, if so, what is it? What Positive Choices is your inner voice urging you to try out or bring forth into your life? If your messenger is silent, it means that you have tuned it out. Start a daily dialogue with this infinite source of wisdom. Write down everything your inner voice is saying, word by word, even if you don't understand what it means. Pay particular attention to any ideas that your messenger has about Positive Choices that will enhance your life.*

Tom kept hearing the words, "Go to the sea; you are meant to live by the sea." Tom was searching for a life partner and had tried personal ads, dating services, fix-ups, and even a matchmaker. When the company he worked for went bankrupt, the messenger became even more insistent. Terrified to move without a job and unsure of what he wanted, he decided to experiment and rented a cottage on a bluff overlooking the Atlantic Ocean for three months, taking advantage of bargain winter-rental rates. His plan was to explore opportunities in the landscaping business and see how he liked a particular resort town and a new lifestyle. It was there he met Bonnie and discovered a niche for his own business as a consultant to national parks.

Tom's messenger had nagged him for more than two years to move to the coast, but it was the trauma of losing his job that paved the way for him actually to try it. Even if this experiment had failed, by acting on his desire to be by the sea, Tom opened himself to learning more about what he truly wanted. Had this particular town not been right, he still would have been armed with new knowledge with which to select his next experiment.

It can be revealing to look at the teachings that come from the languages of other cultures. For example, the Chinese symbol for *crisis* illustrates the interconnection between stress and opportunity. Opportunity can surface disguised as loss, like in Tom's case. His company's financial woes gave him the impetus to pursue his true path. With every problem-solving venture, we gain an opportunity for transformation. Tom discovered new forms of self-expression and contentment by daring to capitalize on his love for the sea and his desire to work outdoors.

To help you to generate even more ideas for Positive Choices to Add to your life, get your journal and find a quiet place to relax where you will not be disturbed. Read through the following exercise and then meditate on it.

INQUIRY *Imagine that you are financially secure and that money is no longer a struggle for you. You are free to use your time in any way you wish and create your life exactly as you desire. Think about all of the things you'd like to do, be, buy, or sample. Don't let you inner critic interrupt this exercise; let your imagination flow freely, ignoring practicality. This is your own private wish list. What opportunities would you welcome into your life? What relationships would you deepen or pursue? What kinds of new people would you like to meet and befriend? What kind of work would be fun and fulfilling for you? Would you work at all and if so, at what? Could your leisure and your work become one? Where would you truly enjoy living? What kind of home would nurture you? What kinds of objects and colors would you surround yourself with? With whom, if anyone, would you live? How would you like to grow personally? What would you most like to learn about? Would you go back to school or create a self-study program? Is traveling part of your fantasy? If so, where and why? How would you like to use your energy in the world? What kind of person would you most like to become? What would make your life meaningful for you? Before you lose the preciousness of these hopes and dreams, jot down anything you want to remember. This Inquiry is a wild-card fantasy designed to connect you with your vision of peak experiences—Positive Choices for you to summon into your life.*

To support the Addition of these opportunities into your life, create or locate visual images of them and compile a Positive Choices collage. Hang it up where you can see it daily.

Chapter 3

S *Is for*
Subtraction

Now that you have declared your priorities
and identified the Positive Choices you want to welcome
into your life, what do you do about the life you have?
How do you deal with the stress levels you feel and the
choices you've made that no longer serve your life story?
Do you feel powerless and out of control of your life?
What's bothering you? All forward movement or growth
begins with letting go. Subtracting unhealthy or negative
life choices that discredit your dreams sends a signal that
you have staked a claim on constructing a better future.

INQUIRY   *What life choices are undermining your
well-being and need to be released? Make a
complete and candid list and then assign an order to
them based on which ones pollute your daily living
the most. These negative life choices are Serenity
Stealers and sabotage your life-force.*

The power of Subtraction is astounding. When we
forcefully say "No" to dysfunctional people, toxic work-
places, limiting beliefs, or unhealthy habits, we open up

the space to fill our lives with what we long for. Is this exchange process easy? No, but this book gives you the tools to manage the process. Sara let go of a graphics business that she had grown to despise and was delighted to find herself re-energized. No longer was she consumed with the politics of making deals or plugging uninspiring products. Now she is flooded with invitations for new social and business connections and is planning a trip around the world to indulge her love of photography. Negative life choices—people, interactions, or situations—siphon your life-force into destructive tributaries and deplete your resources. Save your vitality for the things that really nurture you. Letting go of all the things in your life that don't support you maximizes your precious time. You evolve every day into a new being, and many of the people, projects, and beliefs in your life no longer reflect your emerging self. Deep down, you know what disturbs your inner peace and what you need to cast off.

Your Serenity Stealers function as negative choices, even if you didn't originally select them. What causes you stress is your *relationship* to these Serenity Stealers. It is not your mean-spirited coworker or your noisy street, but your *interaction* with your choices that culminates in negative feelings or responses.

INQUIRY *What are your Serenity Stealers robbing you of? What do they cost you on a physical, psychological, or spiritual level? Is it inner peace, self-*

*respect, or your ability to make good decisions? Be
specific.*

Whenever we grapple with a Serenity Stealer, we have
three options. First of all, we can avoid it. Brendan hates
long commutes, so he always lives and works in close prox-
imity. Spending hours on the expressway with exhausted,
irritable drivers every day, especially in the snow, makes
him anxious. The price of commuting is too high, even
though he's lost out on projects as a result. Look back over
your list of Serenity Stealers and note the ones you can
avoid. Be honest. If your job is horrendous, you could get
another one. If making Thanksgiving dinner for a crowd
totally unnerves you, eat out or get it catered. Too often
our limiting beliefs hypnotize us into thinking we have no
ability to make changes. Stress and stress overload, which
is burnout, often happen when we forget that we do have
ultimate power over our life choices. Once you begin the
process of Subtracting negative choices from your life,
amazing things may happen. Celeste made the agonizing
decision to end her friendship with a woman she had
known since high school. The friend, Dolores, constantly
criticized Celeste's dream to become a teacher and ridiculed
her, saying things like, "You're not interesting enough to
keep people's attention," or "You're not creative enough to
do art with kids." Although Celeste told Dolores on
numerous occasions that her comments were hurtful and
that she was determined to be a great teacher, Dolores continued to undermine her. Finally, Celeste terminated their
relationship. Two weeks later, Celeste met a lovely new

neighbor, a teacher, who helped Celeste with her applications for a master's degree in education and eventually became her mentor. Celeste's clarity that she deserved to have supportive people as friends fine-tuned her criteria for selection.

Your second option when confronting a Serenity Stealer is to alter it. John thought his job as a nurse manager was totally impossible and he would have to quit. Instead he identified his three biggest Serenity Stealers, which were staff shortages, too much paperwork, and the lack of recognition for tasks well done. Proactively, John proposed solutions to each of these morale killers and shared them with his boss. To his surprise, his boss agreed to talk to the board of directors about the feasibility of additional staffing and conceded to let him implement a new software system to streamline the paperwork. Sometimes if we ask, we receive. John now feels more hopeful about an improvement in his work life but is withholding final judgment. If his boss had been unwilling to team up with him and address his complaints, John was ready to resign. Attempts to alter a Serenity Stealer are often worthwhile: even if it doesn't work, the results clarify your next step.

Last, we all encounter Serenity Stealers that we do not have control over. If you contract a serious illness, become the caretaker for an elderly parent, or get sued by a lunatic, you are stuck. But you still have the power to determine how you cope with it. If you are ill, you can research alternative care, locate the best doctors, and find support from other folks with the same diagnosis. If you are a family caretaker, you can enlist aid from other family members, locate community resources, and seek to create the best scenario for all the parties involved. Many adult children actually glean a new closeness with their parents in such a crisis. If you are sued, you can prevent it from happening again and enlist the best legal help you can afford for now. With all of these serious life challenges, you will need to go through a process of analysis to find the right answers. And, rightfully so, you may start out feeling angry and victimized before you can make peace with the hardships you have been dealt. Look for positive role models and ask for support. Seek the lessons hidden in the darkness and leverage them.

Chapter 4

I

Is for
Insight

Feeling resistant yet? Acknowledging that you have the right to Add and Subtract the choices in your life can be a startling concept to absorb. Too often we walk around feeling out of control and abused. We "forget" that we have the power to change most of our circumstances. But psychological resistance may block your willingness to believe that your life can be the way you want it. Insight into your ambivalence or your unwillingness to revitalize your life awakens profound truths.

Tania became clear that she wanted more intimacy and romance from a relationship than existed in her present marriage. Her husband ignored her most of the time and refused to try anything new to spark their passion or friendship. In fact, he told her that if she wasn't happy with the way things were that she ought to leave. For years, Tania had tried to either dazzle him or become indispensable to him. Recently, he became a partner in a high-tech start-up company and had even less time for Tania. After agonizing over his lack of investment in their alliance, Tania got angry. Fueled by the axiom, "Never pursue a distancer," she tried the tactic of becoming unavailable herself. She stayed out late, traveled a lot, and stopped doing his laundry. Her husband seemed oblivious. By now, Tania admitted her defeat but was terrified to Subtract her husband from her life. Why, you might ask, since his lack of caring for her was so apparent? Tania had to admit that she was dependent on him and liked the image of being married, even though she longed to have a deep connection with the right man.

If you find it impossible to let go of a Serenity Stealer, you need to look for insights into the silent payoff. Sometimes a negative choice serves a purpose. We have to discover its hidden meaning before we can move on. For example, if you can never find time to write that novel, you may be protecting yourself from anticipated rejection. You may stay in an intolerable job because you don't want to face the reality that you need to change careers. To admit the underlying payoff for hanging on to negative choices, you must be totally honest with yourself.

To help her get unstuck, Tania completed the following exercise. Try it yourself to illuminate your own reluctance to Subtract what doesn't work in your life, so you can begin again with a Positive Choice.

INQUIRY *Why do you want this negative choice in your life? How does this negative choice serve you? List all of the benefits of settling for this negative choice. Be honest, and write down as many details as you can to help you discover the hidden payoffs. Now, look at how this negative choice pre-*

vents you from growing as a person. How does it undermine your self-esteem and freedom? Finally, try to answer these two questions: Why are you so afraid to let it go? What would it take for you to decide you can release it?

Tania admitted that, although she liked the security of being part of a couple, her husband actually made her feel insecure and undesirable. Yet, Tania feared self-reliance. Staying in this soul-crushing marriage prevented her from exploring her potential. Delving further, Tania realized that the two major ways her husband made her feel cared for were by cooking for her—he was a natural chef— and by managing all the traditional male tasks, like getting the roof repaired and overseeing their expenses and investments. Tania's mother was a businesswoman and, as a child, the family had often eaten take-out food at mealtime, so Tania had little training in kitchen arts. Also, as Tania hadn't worked in years, she had no interest in money nor any idea what her resources were. Tania's insights were that if she could feed herself and manage a checking account, she'd be in a stronger position to consider divorce.

No decision is entirely clear-cut. Tania acknowledged that if she ended her marriage she would miss her in-laws terribly and her vacations at the lake. We have to anticipate that there are losses even in the wisest choices.

Enlisting the support of her friends, Tania signed up for two adult education classes, one in Italian cooking— her favorite style—and a second in financial planning. To her surprise, Tania quickly learned that she was a natural bookkeeper, opened her own checking account, and selected several mutual funds to begin an investment portfolio. After joining an investment club for women, she also got the facts on her assets. Cooking bored her, but she discovered a wonderful gourmet take-out service nearby and elected to invest her energy elsewhere. After several months of independence, Tania committed to her original Positive Choice of securing a better life partner. She bought her own condo near the gourmet shop. She now realized that she had wasted too much time on an unsupportive spouse. Tania Subtracted her husband and created the vacancy for a new partner, and one eventually appeared. Armed with insights and some action steps, Tania overcame her fears and harvested an unknown inner courage. Successful risk-taking fortifies your ability to implement the gains of Addition and Subtraction and continually upgrade your quality of living.

Subtracting a marriage is what I call a "high stakes" change—a major emotional challenge. Some Subtractions, like giving up watching mindless television programs, may be much easier and therefore would be a "low stakes" item. But maybe not. It may be that for you, the television serves as a companion as well as a distraction from your goals, and this issue may generate a monumental dilemma. Classify your potential Subtractions as either high stakes or low stakes in terms of their difficulty for you as an individual. Be prepared for unexpected emotional reactions, like terror or uncertainty, because even positive changes can upset your equilibrium. If you get overwhelmed, back up and see what emotions are ambushing your progress. Ask your inner messenger for help and guidance to accelerate your moving ahead with resolve.

Chapter 5

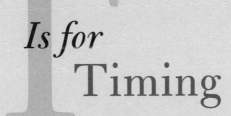

Is for
Timing

Selecting life changes to tackle and then timing the changes are two key factors in your decision-making process. Choices are complex—that's why it's best to start with easy Subtractions. Resigning from a committee is much less challenging than researching new careers or other choices that involve risks, experiments, and inevitable failures on the path to your goal. To help you to determine an appropriate plan for your Additions and Subtractions, you need to assess your available physical and psychological energy levels. Even the most positive of changes requires adaptation and readjustment and therefore demands your energy.

INQUIRY *How much available energy do you have for one or more transitions this year? Make a list of key events that have happened to you already this calendar year. Did you change jobs or your standard of living? Begin or end a relationship? Care for a sick relative? Lose your best friend? Find out you have high blood pressure? In sum, has it been an eventful year for you? Add up the number of changes you* *have processed this year and then rate them in terms of the intensity of their energy drain on your body, mind, and spirit.*

Are you feeling burned out—like you can't handle another new challenge? If the challenges of a normal day regularly make you want to bury yourself in your comforter, you may be burned out from too much change. You need time to reflect and integrate what's already happened to you. Or are you ready to scream from boredom? If you are eager for new beginnings or ready to unload the things that just don't resonate with your new life plan, engaging with change is a Positive Choice for you now. Or is your experience mixed? For example, Joe bought a new house that he loves, but he also feels ambivalent about the maintenance required every weekend.

Try to assign a percentage to how much free energy you have for something new. Paula spent the past year moving her mother to a nursing home, selling the family home, and fighting with her siblings over who got the family silver. She took good care of herself during this stressful time, so she estimated that she had about 75 percent of her physical energy available to move ahead. But, psychologically, she felt "fried" and needed time to heal from all of the trauma; she rated herself as only 20 percent available for change. So, instead of moving herself and her business to a new location as planned, she determined that the only Addition she wanted to add in for the next three months was to join a dream group. Everything else needed to wait until she recouped her psychological stamina. Think about what, based on your reserves, you could handle during the next twelve months.

INQUIRY *Are there either Additions or Subtractions that you want to manifest this year that need to be postponed? Which do you have the desire to handle now and which options feel overwhelming or less imperative? When you've identified what you'd like to postpone, ask yourself if this is a healthy, life-enhancing postponement or a daunting procrastination. Positive postponements are another form of Subtraction. Acts of procrastination need to be analyzed truthfully and then either be eliminated, delegated, or given top priority. If it is a healthy postponement, then pull out a calendar and choose a month to reconsider this issue.*

Now that you have realistically assessed which choices you can manage now and which choices need to be postponed, you can prioritize your high-stakes and low-stakes Subtractions to help determine the best timing for you. Sometimes we go through life-cycles in which everything is a struggle or is fraught with roadblocks. If you are in the midst of one of these cycles where nothing is evolving easily, your timing may be off. Life-cycles, like creativity cycles, run in circles of birth, decay, death, and rebirth. Think about the current context in which you are operating. Mike's architecture business floundered for years with extreme swings in projects and income. But over the past year, even though the real estate market in his area has stayed about the same, he's finally getting the clients he wants, and things seem easy all of a sudden. He's immersed in a flow cycle in his life and feels more confident about making more daring Additions and Subtractions. Are you in a period of success or a period of stagnation? Being aware of which kind of backdrop you are experiencing arms you with additional information to help you make good decisions about timing.

INQUIRY *Of all of the Serenity Stealers that you want to Subtract, which one will most dramatically improve the ambiance of your life when it is gone? Do you have the energy to Subtract that negative life choice now? When is the best time for you to begin? If you are not ready to change this highest-stakes item, what can you Subtract now instead? Keep asking yourself these questions on a monthly basis to create a momentum of Subtractions in your life until you have cleared out the bulk of your Serenity Stealers.*

Unfortunately, you will continue to confront new Serenity Stealers, but one hopes that they will be easier to delete. The open space in your life can now be filled with those coveted Positive Choices, carefully selected in a timely fashion. Identifying your personal timing patterns ensures greater success with your initiations of life changes.

Chapter 6

I

Is for
Invitation

I

Invitation is about welcoming support systems into your life to promote the likelihood of your triumph with your Addition and Subtraction exchanges. Reviewing your previous Inquiries, select a priority list of five Positive Choices you want to Add to your life and five Serenity Stealers you want to Subtract. They can be either high- or low-stakes items, but make sure they are the first ones you want to engage with. Even if you have chosen to postpone the actual exchange due to low energy, follow along with us so you will be extra-prepared when you are ready to move ahead. Aside from these ten choices, be sure to keep track of your other options on a backlist and save them for future reference.

Let's begin with your Subtraction List. Are there any items on the list that are easy and could be completed today? Clark had been grieving a relationship with a woman who left him. He knew he needed to let go of her completely but still had a photo collection of their good times displayed in his den. Removing those pictures was a big Subtraction for him. But finally he knew he was ready and dumped those photos into the trash compactor. If you're prepared to Subtract something today, give it a try.

When you practice discarding easier items, you will be more prepared to release the harder Serenity Stealers on your list. If you can't complete the Subtraction process now, at least you started the action mode.

While there may be a few things that can be easily disposed of, many Serenity Stealers can be extremely challenging. Think now about one of the more difficult Serenity Stealers on your list. To help you to get a clear handle on the real issues behind your Serenity Stealer, you need to dig a little deeper into your resistance.

INQUIRY *What's your attachment to this Serenity Stealer? Write a pro and con list for this choice, as if you hadn't ever decided to have it in your life.*

To help you to identify the particulars of the Serenity Stealer you want to eliminate, you must study it. The additional information will support your efforts.

INQUIRY *Keep a detailed diary about this Serenity Stealer for two weeks. Be as specific as possible and brainstorm unconventional solutions to your dilemma. Sometimes limited thinking can be the worst Serenity Stealer of all. Use the five Ws: What, Where, When, Why, and Whom. Also log your emotional and physical reactions about how you cope. Think about whether this choice needs to be totally eliminated or can simply be modified, including changing your attitude about it to reduce its impact.*

Last, see if you can discover the most compelling issue you must resolve to release your Serenity Stealer.

Careful study should bring the truth to the surface. If not, tell your story to a trusted ally and get an objective view. Awareness is the first step in the change process. At the end of two weeks, your dilemma will be clearer. Once you have at least a hypothesis, make a Subtraction plan you can live with and implement it. If it doesn't work, revise it again. Write in your journal every day why you *don't* want this choice anymore. You will release it when you are finished with its lessons.

Part of the Invitation process is seeking support from strategies that reflect your personality and personal style as well as from people who can assist you. Think about whether or not you need a mentor, a support group, a coach, or a counselor to help you either to get unstuck or to launch you forward faster and further. How about a class, a workshop, a book, or a video to inspire or educate you in new ways of doing things? Is it time to wrestle with your spiritual beliefs and find the ideology you rely on? Is it time to hire help, delegate, or invent a new model of Subtraction for yourself? You need support to withstand the trials of change and the urge to cop out. Asking for help and identifying your model of support increases your chances for success. You will also feel less alone and build a new skill set in the process.

Another aspect of Invitation is the power of declaration and intention. When you decide to set boundaries in your life and to no longer tolerate a Serenity Stealer, the universe supports that intention. Subtraction, or your willingness to consider Subtraction, engages unknown gifts and often speeds up the cycle of attracting those Positive Choices you really want in your life. Trevor was amazed at what happened after he declared his intention to get promoted to vice president at his company or leave. All of a sudden, he met a new mentor in the lunchroom, got permission to go to an expensive management- development conference, and discovered two books on team building in the "New Nonfiction" section of his local library. The universe was signaling to him that pursuing this promotion was the right path for now.

Synchronicities and chance meetings that propel us forward support our wisely chosen Positive Choices and our new lives. Open up to these wonderful bonuses. Declare your desire for support and new connections to fuel your creative process. So you don't get too complacent or miss the benevolence, keep a list of these events, and be grateful. Also recognize that you may go through a period where your commitment will be tested. Watch for both tricks and pitfalls in your change evolution. Avoid all persons who do not support your growth; they are treacherous as well.

Chapter 7

V
Is for
Visualization

Part of reinventing your life is increasing your comfort level with acquiring your Positive Choices Additions. When you are beckoning Additions into your life, visualization is a powerful preparation tool. When you stake a claim on a more favorable future, you have to wrestle with the discomfort of change. The purpose of doing your Positive Choices collage (chapter 2) was to implant vivid pictures of your Additions into your consciousness. But visualization actually gives you a dress rehearsal of your new role. The power of visualization is that it allows you to practice being in your desired state. It also facilitates the release of your belief that you can't have what you want. By using compelling images in a visualization, you cancel out your fears and increase your receptivity to the steps of manifestation.

INQUIRY *Set aside a quiet time to visualize your ideal life of Positive Choices. Find a comfortable seat in your home or office, turn off the phone, and get ready to visualize your new life. Light a candle or place some spiritual symbols of comfort around you.*

Put your Positive Choices collage and your lists of Additions and Subtractions in front of you. Study the details of your collage and your lists. Close your eyes and relax. Simply let go of all stress and worry and tune into the excitement of re-creating your life. Zero in on your Subtraction list, wrap it in a white cloud, and send those Serenity Stealers away into the atmosphere. You have banished them and created open space instead. Get a clear picture of your life with the Addition of your Positive Choices. Let them appear in your vision, one by one. Picture a perfect day enjoying these Additions, noticing their nuances and influence on you. Imagine that they precipitate your personal transformation. Memorize the feelings of contentment associated with experiencing this new life of Positive Choices. Spend ten minutes a day getting increasingly cozy with your newly empowered self, and open your eyes when you feel complete.

Because visualization is a preview of what you choose to create, write down everything you can remember from your visual experience. Sometimes you will get an inkling about modifying your vision. For example, one of Marcy's Positive Choices was her wish to run a home-based wedding floral business. She loved the idea that she could work whenever she chose and planned to convert her basement into a storage area for ribbons and supplies and install giant refrigerators in her garage. In the midst of her fourth visualization, Marcy pictured customers all over her house and realized that she had neglected to consider her great love of privacy. The next day she tried her visualization with her business located in a shop in the center of town. This new vision clicked. She began to look for retail space and redid her business plan accordingly.

Visualization also helps to illuminate unconscious fears or conflicts in anticipation of your new life. Bob and his wife were unable to have children, so they planned to adopt a baby from China. They had been approved by an agency and now were just waiting. Parenting a child was Bob's number 1 most important Addition on his list. Yet, the first time he visualized himself alone holding his adopted child, he dropped her onto the floor—accidentally. He opened his eyes feeling terrified about making mistakes as a parent and unintentionally hurting this fragile, vulnerable baby girl. He talked his fears over with his wife, and together they decided to take a parenting course offered at their local hospital that covered the basics of baby care. This class, combined with conversations with parents that he admired, toned down his fears. His visualizations progressed to images of him happily playing with his new baby and the two of them laughing and bonding. Shortly after he resolved these fears, they got the call to fly to China to pick up their daughter-to-be. Bob felt truly ready now.

Visualization dynamites away your limiting beliefs. Every day that you picture yourself abundant with your new Positive Choices, you relinquish any attachment to suffering and struggle. This doesn't mean that you may not have to work hard to attain your dreams. But suffering and struggle can render the process all the more draining and disheartening. Settling for less than we can have is another characteristic of limiting our potential. Sara wanted a marketing consulting assignment that would pay her bills, stimulate her ability to generate new ideas, and allow her to travel to lovely places a few times a year. In the wake of one of her visualizations, surprisingly, she saw herself as an equity partner in a new e-commerce venture where her marketing strategies directly catapulted the company to success. All of a sudden, she realized that there was the possibility of real wealth from such an assignment. She could potentially make several million dollars from the venture. As the work tapped into her greatest skills, it was easy and pleasurable for her to reap these extraordinary benefits. Her visualizations helped her to believe it was indeed possible and that she could handle becoming the wealthy woman she never expected to be. In one of her visualizations, she saw herself funding a new multimedia library in her community. This image fueled her passion to forge ahead, capture this amazing opportunity, and in turn, share her good fortune with others.

Your Positive Choices are catalysts for adding more drama and self-expression to your life and the lives of all that you touch. By trying them on ahead of time to ensure that the fit and comfort levels are accurate, you have the opportunity to refine and expand your dreams from the safety of your armchair. In addition, you are telegraphing to the universe that you intend to live this unique new life that you can now see so clearly.

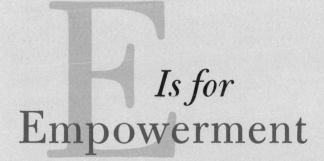

Chapter 8

Is for
Empowerment

The biggest obstacle in this experiment of quality living is often yourself. You have to *believe* it is possible to feel more centered and fulfilled, or it will never happen. You also need the strength and faith to hang on when your visions don't manifest or if they take longer than you expected. Sometimes holdups may signal that your plan is off target or that you are getting in your own way. During these times of delay or confusion, be sure to invite the support of your fellow "travelers" on the Positive Choices path—you'll be better able to stay confident and keep trying.

Choosing the bridge of Positive Choices was an act of empowerment. It is further empowering to be armed with self-knowledge about your patterns of success and failure, so that when you tackle difficult Subtractions or endeavor to accept the rightness of your Additions, you know your history of strengths and weaknesses. You will then be better able to choose what attributes you have to either leverage or overcome.

Identify the Additions or Subtractions on your list of ten that you anticipate having the most difficulty with. By projecting ahead and identifying the potential obstacles, you increase your chances of victory.

INQUIRY *Focusing on one Addition or Subtraction that you feel anxious about, ask yourself the following questions: What strategies have I tried so far, and why haven't they worked? Do I have any personal barriers to overcome first? (Possible personal barriers to success might include trying to solve the wrong problem, procrastinating, not taking responsibility for your contribution to a problem, giving up too easily, putting others' needs first, not asking for help, not being clear about what you want, or having unrealistic expectations of yourself or others.) Do I need to learn some new skills to resolve my situation? If so, what are they and how can I get them? What kinds of support systems would increase my success potential? What decisions can I make today and put into action that will help resolve this situation? Write down your responses and start to make things happen. If you are not successful, go through this list again and try once more.*

Karl wanted to indulge his love of music by composing and then selling a popular song. However, he continually failed to get beyond the starting point. He had written a few lines but became easily distracted from his goal. Karl felt exasperated with his lack of progress. He pondered the empowerment questions and began to recognize how he was ducking the difficulties. He realized that most of his successes in life had resulted from responding to firm deadlines and feeling informed. Writing and selling a song was too open-ended a task for him and far too easy to postpone. Also, when he sat down at the piano, he never got beyond the first few lines because he felt blocked. He quit too soon and never resolved his composition dilemmas. In addition, he'd never taken a music-writing course, an experience that would increase his skill and confidence levels and also help him get accustomed to working with composition deadlines. Karl also realized that if anyone else was in the house, he wasn't able to write at home. So Karl signed up for a course and also arranged to go into his day job a few hours later two days a week so that he could enjoy quiet time while members of his family were at work or school.

Another obstacle for Karl was his lack of knowledge about the copyright process and his concern about people stealing his ideas. So he networked his way to a creative-arts lawyer and got a consultation on the details of the copyright process.

Each of these steps broke through his impasse. Karl visualized completing his song within six months, and he did. He then hired an agent who introduced him to a wonderful small recording company. By the end of two years, Karl had completed a full CD. By acknowledging the truth about how he operated, Karl was able to become empowered, triumph over his obstacles, and move up to the next level of success.

Use your visualization exercises to try on new behaviors and see whether they achieve the results you want. Belle's vision was to become physically fit and strong so that she could enjoy hiking with her family and friends. In her fifty-two years of living, Belle had never been athletic and had never sustained a workout program for more than several months. Insights into her personal style inspired her to design a working plan. She determined that she was incapable of self-directing her fitness program. So she did three things: hired a personal trainer, joined a lovely fitness club with a great restaurant, and enrolled in a healthy heart program at her local hospital with classes and medical checkups. Her friends all told her that this was major overkill and that her muscles would be screaming in pain from all of this exercise. She assured them that she would alternate exercises. Belle also reserved a hiking lodge in the Rockies for herself and her family six months into the future. She was committed like never before. What Belle knew was that, for her, exercise had to be social, so she purposely connected with numerous people in her three fitness programs.

She completed her hospital program of ten weeks, volunteered to run the daily walking groups at her health club, and continued with her personal trainer at home. The Rockies trip happened as well. Belle set up the next family hiking trip two days after she came home, just to keep the momentum going. By leveraging her personality as a natural leader and someone who keeps her commitments to others, Belle set up a structure that ensured that her personal fitness became a group project. While her body felt stronger, it was her relationships with people, not better health, that sustained her actions. By having to show up to lead a walking group every day, she walked whether she felt like it or not, because the group depended on her. By studying her failures in the past, Belle designed her current plan to reflect her value system.

Empower yourself by reviewing your strengths and weaknesses and determining what motivates you to implement a lasting change. Then push yourself to that next precipice.

part II

The
Power *of*
Choices

Congratulations! You have made it to part two of the Positive Choices journey. Now, using the seven letters in the word *Choices,* you will create an expanded list of Positive Choices and learn additional practices to maximize your ability to attain the life you have imagined so far.

Choosing is a dramatic action. It says Yes to a life decision as well as No to a less desirable option. The choices you make in your life express who you are and reflect your originality. Your life choices mirror your personality, preferences, intuitions, dreams, and idiosyncrasies.

Choosing your life circumstances heralds the life you envision. It also affirms that you *do* have freedom of choice. Within that entitlement, you can discern which choices you welcome into your life experience and which ones you cancel out. Happy, contented people make conscious, careful choices about their life focuses that endorse their individual values. Choosing proclaims your personal power.

Chapter 9

Is for
Centering

It is vital that you employ strategies to keep you centered while you are blazing new life pathways. The novelty of Additions and Subtractions can cause you to feel adrift at sea without an anchor. You need your anchors during times of transition so that you can feel grounded and on an even keel.

INQUIRY *What are your personal anchors—people, things, places, or rituals—that keep you connected to yourself, your sense of well-being, and your feelings? What makes you feel secure in the world? Who or what can you count on for support? What comforts you when you feel unnerved? Make a list of these anchors so you can access them when you feel stranded and unsure.*

Inner stillness serves as a powerful anchor. Quiet is incredibly healing. Turn off the voices of outsiders, and listen to your own sacred thoughts and feelings. Or listen to the wind, the rain, or the sea. Feel your connection with them and the universe. Or simply relax and don't think; instead, tune into your groundedness in the Earth—your connection with all that has come before and will follow you.

When you are depleted, you have nothing to share with anyone else. Take extra time for yourself. Find a way to carve out the time. Leave work early, take a long lunch, trade baby-sitting favors with a friend or spouse, or brainstorm support options with a group of friends. In order to build a better life, you must take this respite time daily to integrate all of the internal and external changes. Silence lets you hear your own genius. Quiet gives you space to breathe and linger at a slower pace. Centering yourself daily will protect your loved ones as well. Many people unintentionally—and with great regret—respond to chaos by becoming irritable or irrational with the people they care about the most. The stress that comes from adjusting to life changes—even ones that are wonderful for you—has to be siphoned off somewhere. If you find yourself picking on people or being short-fused, retreat into your own space and sort it out.

INQUIRY *Are you actually upset with the person(s) that you feel angry or disturbed with? Or are you suffering from the stress of change and your inability to manage it? Separate out the issues that are your own from those that are related to the people you care for and that need to be resolved with them. Rectify your own issues first. After you've*

*done that, you'll be in a better space to negotiate
with your loved ones or colleagues.*

Alert the people you are in partnership or relationship
with that you are forging ahead with new goals and may
show some signs of disorientation. Let them know as well
that you may need an unusual amount of time by yourself
to process the pluses and minuses of each Addition and
Subtraction. Time alone allows you to dissect the real
dilemmas and take your emotional temperature. It also
increases the likelihood that you will be able to relate
more authentically to others and grow those relationships
as well. If you are a parent, don't sacrifice everything for
your children. Try to model mutuality and balance, so
your children will do the same in their future relationships. Staying connected to your thoughts and emotions
ensures that you will maintain strong relationships with
the right people who support your new life choices.

Some form of creative arts can also be a superb centering tool for your transition. Marcus carved a series of
wood sculptures to represent several leisure options for
his retirement. As a devoted workaholic, he knew that his
forced early retirement could be troublesome. He kept
hearing about men dying in the first year after retirement,
and he didn't want to abandon his family in this way. So
his intuition urged him to try woodcarving. With great
thoughtfulness, he produced a series of carvings of a fish-
erman, a philanthropist, a ski instructor, and a business
advisor. This collection helped Marcus to try on new
identities by intensely pondering each one.

Jeannette kept a journal detailing the drama of her battle to Subtract her shopaholic lifestyle and become financially secure. She wrote in great detail about cutting up her credit cards, doing volunteer work instead of shopping on Saturdays, and having a series of yard sales to unload previous purchases. Her journal read like a roller coaster of hope and despair and included disguised renderings from her Debtors' Anonymous meetings. The Subtraction of her shopping addiction consumed her until she untangled her childhood attachments to money. Jeannette's gift for humor glimmered through the pages of her journal. Her inner voice chimed in one day and urged her to write a play about her trial with debt. She's working on it. Sharing her story with others will help her to stay centered herself. Your creative self can help you record your progress, highlighting your gains and losses. By recording or representing your musings, new perceptions emerge.

Both time alone and creative arts can help you to build a stronger bond with your intuitive voice of wisdom and guidance. A key benefit of centering is magnifying your own opinions and hunches. Do you have lots of voices rattling around in your head? You have many parts to yourself—your internal critic, your impulsive self, and your voice of reason. Your intuitive voice links together your other voices to create fresh ideas for you.

Can you recall a time when your intuitive voice advised you not to do something and you didn't listen? Bob remembers being at a job interview with the woman who would be his boss; his intuitive voice kept urgently whispering to him, "She's a liar and a phony." Bob was sick of job hunting, so he stifled his intuitive voice and accepted the job. Within two weeks, his intuition was confirmed: his new boss was not trustworthy.

Your inner wisdom can become a cherished advisor when you take the time to get acquainted with that voice. Play with runes, tarot cards, or other self-awareness tools and learn about the splendor of your internal workings and insights. Once you trust your own wisdom, your path to serenity will be smoother. Fine-tune your senses. Observe the beauty of Nature, art, and the world around you. When you feel stuck on a problem, go look at a flower—or any other object in Nature—and pay attention to its every detail and nuance. That flower will trigger new metaphors and connections and potentially will generate new solutions.

Think about how you feel when you listen to your favorite music. What else energizes you? What photographs, paintings, or posters inspire you? What pulls you down? Throw out anything that doesn't excite you or touch you deeply. Surround yourself with colors and environments that nourish you. When you buy something, ask yourself, "Does it make my heart sing?" If not, pass it by. Mediocrity dulls the senses. Rediscover your own tastes and make them part of your everyday experience. Centering yourself enhances your ability to accomplish your intentions, allowing your emotions to help you to avoid pitfalls and ditches along the way. Let your healing need for tranquility—including people, environments, and activities that steady your equilibrium—create an inner strength that will solidly ground you regardless of the challenges you decide to tackle.

Chapter 10

H

Is for
Honoring

Honoring your unique self in life gives you an edge. Uncovering the real truth about your personal style and your preferences allows you to create a lifestyle that's in alignment with who you really are—not the person someone else urged you to be. Part of your Subtraction process needs to be deleting other people's expectations and agendas for your life. By Subtracting their scripts for you, you can write your own screenplay, choosing every detail, including only Additions that you love. Carefully evaluate which life choices nourish you and which ones deplete your sense of well-being. Those insights are the gems from which you craft your original life episodes.

INQUIRY *Are you following someone else's casting call? Are you an artist at heart dressed up in a suit? Or a country soul living in a high-rise studio apartment? Have you made lifestyle choices because you were supposed to? What parts of yourself are you not honoring? Release your attachment to other people's approval and set yourself free to select only the Positive Choices that are best for you.*

Brian gave up his investment banking career because he wanted to get to know his children, something his high-powered father never did. After Brian's twins were born, being a great father became more important than his original career dreams of acquiring wealth for himself and his clients. It took a lot of courage for Brian to break the family tradition of three generations of male investment bankers. But he had vivid memories of waiting up for his dad to come home from work and falling asleep before he arrived. He remembers wishing that his dad could watch him play soccer on Saturdays or help him with his homework. Brian's childhood was very lonely, and he admits that he always doubted whether his father really loved him. As a young child, Brian vowed to himself that if he were ever a dad, he'd never make his children suffer that way. Honoring his youthful promise to himself, Brian resigned from his top New York firm and instead selected a position in a regional bank with reasonable hours and a fifteen-minute commute. He also became the coach for his kids' sports teams as well as the family cook. While he missed his old luxuries at times, he felt proud of the man he had chosen to become.

Myrna spent years trying to be a corporate trainer even though she knew in her heart that it was too extroverted a career choice for her. She fell into it, though, and the money was great. Her dad was a professor and her mom was a stockbroker, so her role models were big talkers and storytellers. Although Myrna prepared diligently and received great evaluations from her classes, she felt exhausted by being "on" all the time. When a training recession hit, Myrna had some time to rethink her choice. She longed for a quieter, more low-key life behind the scenes, one that honored her introverted being. She wanted to be in charge of her own schedule and her own thoughts. Training involved too much performing and people contact. She's now an instructional designer based at home and is quite content.

Don't wait till a midlife crisis occurs to claim what you want. Is your life too stressful? Perhaps you are pushing yourself in the wrong direction. Ever notice how some things just work easily and others are a constant pain? There may be some clues there. Your own Positive Choices mirror who you are. Rework your life around them.

Also, honor the signals from your body. What tells you when you need to exercise, make love, or see a doctor? We're not talking hypochondria here—just awareness. Burnout often continues when you don't heed your body's demands for vacations or something new. Jason knows that when his left eye starts to twitch, he's in trouble. It means there's an internal struggle he's not dealing with. His twitchy eye alerts him to take action. So, he makes a dinner date with the person who knows him best—an old college buddy, John—and they ferret out his conflict. John calls him a few months later, when there's a problem he wants to talk over.

Laura frequently has pain in her neck muscles. That's a clue for her to stop and lie down. Often the pain occurs when she's mad at her husband and needs to balance her anger with her affection for him. It is wise to heed these less serious symptoms and learn their lessons. Don't ignore them and wait for a more serious wake-up call, like a heart attack. Your body is another messenger in your repertoire, so gratefully honor its wisdom.

INQUIRY *How is your body feeling? What tensions, abnormalities, or discomforts are disturbing you? Try to notice when these symptoms occur and what might precipitate them. Don't blame yourself for any physical ailments. Simply make the time to notice them, and then get the care you need—be it physical, emotional, or medical—to be sure that you are living the best possible life you can to keep yourself healthy.*

Self-honor dramatically improves your ability to make the right Additions and Subtractions to ensure your fulfillment. I often hear artists say that they wish they could just be accountants, as life would be so much easier. If you are a true artist, it is unlikely that you'd be happy as an accountant. Trying to be a "numbers person" is actually harder for an artist than capitalizing on a love of color and beauty. Honor who you truly are, and life will be smoother. You increase your chances of prosperity when you play to your best aptitudes.

Chapter 11

Is for
Owning

Have you forsaken a creative wish that once meant a lot to you? Reclaiming the lost dreams of adolescence and childhood re-energizes you! Juan switched majors in college from interior design to business because his advisor thought it was a more practical course of study. While his finance classes were interesting, he was much more drawn to the worlds of architecture and antiques. After college, he became a prestigious high-technology executive but felt disconnected from his work and the products. When his company moved, he redecorated his home and faced the facts. He still wanted to be a designer. A certification program later, Juan now works at an upscale retailer.

As a child, Sherry used to play endlessly with LEGOs. She knew that building things was her dream. But dollar signs beckoned her toward a lucrative career in advertising, and she excelled. After ten years, she confessed to a friend that she hated the work, the travel, and the impersonal nature of the business. She quit and started over. Today she is a general contractor and constructs gorgeous sunrooms for homes and offices. Both Juan and Sherry originally opted for paths of economic security, and misery led them back to their true callings. Own your desires and impulses.

INQUIRY *Do you have flashes of inspiration? Are you capturing them? Are you expressing them? Do you dismiss your innovative thoughts out of fear? What is the source of that fear—your family, your teachers, your workplace? Creative thinking requires courage and practice. Resolve to add some Positive Choices to help you to forge ahead. What would you like to try?*

Sudi always loved the idea of farming and fantasized about owning a Christmas tree farm one day. While she had lots of lush plants in her indoor urban garden, she knew nothing about the specifics of tree farming on a commercial level. She decided to get a job at a nursery in the suburbs, working with the owner and his children, who had all grown up with dirt and seedlings. Early on, Sudi racked up some embarrassing moments and stumbled through that first planting season. On her drives home from the nursery, with all ten fingernails broken and scratches all over her arms, Sudi wondered if her dream was insane. Yet, the learning fascinated her, and she loved seeing the tiny trees covered in snow the following winter. Fortunately, Sudi's determination and love of nature are spurring her onward. She consciously owns her interests, and finding land in Vermont lures her now.

When was the last time you took a picture or fashioned a costume or told a joke? Notice what you long to express. What are the things that you are intrigued by but talk yourself out of doing? Find some folks who've stayed on the track you're interested in, and get their advice about how to make your dream into reality. So often in our culture, creative dreams are easily dismissed as foolish.

Impress yourself first. Let go of public pretense. All for show? What an empty way to live. When people are faced with dying, they often take off the shackles of propriety and declare their independence. What compromises are you making in your life because it "looks good" to your parents, your coworkers, or your neighbors? Internal conflicts often occur because you don't totally accept who you are. Positive Choices help you to express your real self—what satisfies and inspires you. When you express a false self, you miss your spiritual connection with others as well as yourself. What are you doing simply for approval from others? Bob dislikes yard work, and it irritates his sinuses. He realized that he was afraid that his neighbors would think he was uppity if he hired a landscaper. Then he realized that paying a landscaper was cheaper than expensive allergist appointments and medications. So he Subtracted his yard work in order to take care of himself and hired Lovely Landscapes. Owning his own needs became a higher priority than pleasing the neighbors. And the landscaper, of course, appreciated the work. So often when we delegate, others benefit.

INQUIRY *As you read along, be sure and capture any new Additions and Subtractions that you want to add to your master list. Are you still pursuing the right goals or are they shifting somewhat? Do your goals need fine-tuning or reconsideration? Pay attention to the nuances of new perceptions as they emerge.*

What is fascinating about the quest for a life filled with glorious Positive Choices is noting your evolution into a more authentic human being. By embracing life choices that mirror your personal priorities and values, you feel more like yourself than ever and know that finally, you are in charge of your life!

Chapter 12

I

Is for
Inventing

I

Inventing a new life reflects your capacity for innovation. So many midlifers simply long to enjoy their lives more, tapping into that childhood wonder of fun and adventure.

INQUIRY *When was the last time you truly had fun? Do you know what fun is for you? What brings joy to your heart and draws you into the moment? Is your work pleasurable, or would you give it up in a minute and sail around the world? What gets you out of bed in the morning these days?*

People are often their most imaginative when they are at play or just fooling around with new thoughts. How much of your life do you spend in the fun mode? Back in the '70s, you could earn a master's degree in leisure counseling. The futurists at that time were certain that automation would create three-day work weeks and therefore an abundance of leisure time. That was a faulty prediction. In this international economy, work hours have increased and vacations have gotten shorter. Yet, leisure as play is indeed a science of rejuvenation and recovery. When you fill your life with Positive Choices related to recreation—which means re-creation—you sample another dimension of yourself.

Tim had a longtime urge to fly a kite. He finally went into a kite store and picked out a snazzy eagle model. Several months later, he drove to a field in the country to launch it. His first flight was a success. Tim then began collecting unusual bird kites. One day he realized that his kites were a metaphor for possibilities—an antidote to limited thinking. He began to share his kites with friends and sponsored kite-flying day trips to challenging places with steep cliffs and lots of wind. His spirit of adventure and creativity flowed, and he became known as the kite man. Your playfulness has much to teach you if you let it emerge!

Another key part of inventiveness is letting in the unexpected from others. I call it "gracious receiving." Stop putting out for a moment, and let the universe reciprocate. Observe the input/output balance in your life. If you feel drained from doing too much or trying too hard, it's time to shift the balance. Do you turn down offers of help? Do you feel uncomfortable delegating to someone else? Do you take over tasks that truly belong to another person?

Catie tried an experiment. She felt angry at her family because they didn't help enough around the house—she ended up doing everything. So she went on strike for a week. She didn't shop, cook, pick up, wash, or nag. No one seemed to notice for a few days. All of a sudden they said, "What's going on?" Catie realized that she obviously had higher standards and finished everything before the rest of the family even noticed that it needed to be done. So she called a family meeting and they began a new experiment—jobs for everyone. Letting go is essential to receiving.

To inspire your inventive energy, you need to banish the *shoulds* in your life. Stress relief is about perception. When you feel you *should* do something, you may feel a joylessness about it. When you shift your focus to *wanting* to do something, your whole experience is transformed. *Wanting* implies choosing.

INQUIRY *Make a list of obligations, responsibilities, or entanglements that feel burdensome to you. Now imagine "wanting" to do these tasks and note how your attitude shifts as a result.*

Should is a classic Serenity Stealer. It's a setup for suffering and deprivation. It also has a parental tone, which implies work. Notice the difference when you say, "I should read my child a story at bedtime," versus "I want to read our favorite story *The Velveteen Rabbit* with my child tonight." The energy in your body is much lighter with the "want" option, isn't it?

After all, most of us can generate a list of *shoulds* that would take a lifetime to complete. We subscribe to the illusion that once everything's done, we will be calm. This kind of tranquility is a seductive but unattainable state. So remind yourself to stay in the moment and choose what you are doing. The *shoulds* can be harnessed. Does your office need to be reorganized? Pretend you are an anthropologist; take an excursion to an office supply store, and play with the array of gadgets out there. Are there new multifunction telephones or online filing software or color-coded file cards that will entice you to stay streamlined? Enjoy the discovery process and choose items that could potentially resolve your personal time-management pitfalls. Make a game out of it as opposed to flogging yourself for being disorganized. The mind-set of *wanting* an efficient workspace allows you to delight in the escapade of it.

Carlos noticed that he felt burdened by his To Do list, because he could never get to the end of it. He routinely set humanly impossible expectations for himself. So he shortened it to no more than ten items per day so that he could go at a more leisurely pace and revel in each activity. To accomplish this, he subtracted lots of *shoulds*. Don't set yourself up for failure—try a new technique instead.

Susannah bought an old Victorian home with gingerbread windows, a wraparound porch, and lots of secret corners for her cat to hide in. The only surprise about the house was the large number of minor repairs it required. She dreaded taking doors off hinges and changing window locks. So she got inventive and made a deal with her neighbor Justin, who was a single parent. He works as her handyman, and, in exchange, she watches his children after school two days a week. Now she has time to make tea and sit in her rocker on the porch and play with the cat. Joyful moments—they're priceless.

Put a *J* for joy on your To Do list today next to the items that you're looking forward to. Then see what you can do to change your experience of the rest. You want to languish in the wonder of planting your geraniums, not suffer through it. Think of all the precious moments that are lost to you because you are cramming them into an already overloaded day.

Tune in to yourself a few times a day and ask, "Am I having a good time? What can I do to make today more pleasurable for myself and others?" Suffering is not the purpose of living. See if emphasizing your need for pleasure increases its presence in your life. Unleash your inventiveness to elevate your life to an art form. Did you love your shower today?

Chapter 13

C

Is for
Committing

Committing to taking calculated, healthy risks will advance your goals. Transforming your life with Positive Choices demands commitment and the courage to compose a life that reflects your needs, values, and loves. Committing to your course of action and surviving the trials of change is essential.

Kerry was petrified to let go of her successful biotechnology career, but she truly wanted to pursue her own research in immunology and mentor graduate students at a university. Trading a $90,000 salary for a $40,000 one—even with the likely possibility of consulting contracts—takes guts. Her family supported her in her move to academia, but her biotechnology colleagues thought she was foolish. A year later, Kerry is happier, her family relishes having her home nearly every night for dinner, and she has a patent pending on a formula. She will probably end up ahead financially.

The invitation to be entrepreneurial and generate your own work and family constellations is becoming a trend. Giving up the guarantee of security is scary and calls upon your inner resources. Committing to the plan you want is key. The Greeks say that the word *risk* means "to sail around a cliff." It is a journey into the unknown and the unknowable that challenges your faith and self-confidence. Risks, especially calculated ones, fertilize your growth and stretch your internal workings in new directions.

Yet risks need to be carefully considered. Risks should not endanger you or your loved ones or your basic needs. Take in the encouragement of other Positive Choices seekers, and surround yourself with people who have your best interests at heart. At the same time, consider the value of the warnings from the "Keep the status quo at all costs" types without being pulled into unnecessary negativity.

INQUIRY *Who supports you in this risk and who doesn't? Can you find benefit in the counsel on both sides of the issue? Interview people who have done what you are trying to do. Soak up their advice, assuming they are supportive and not competitive. There's nothing like expert advice from those who've been there already.*

Make sure that you have the desire and ability to do what it takes to achieve your goals. If you want to be the spokesperson for an organization, get some public speaking training and/or media coaching so that you can effectively communicate your message to large numbers of people. If you need capital to start a business, find out the most clever and compelling ways to attract investors. If you don't have the skills or interest to prepare your case, hire others to fortify your project so that you get the financial support you require. Again, listen to your adversaries to see what you can learn from them, but gather into your inner circle people who believe in your mission and intention.

INQUIRY *With your risk in mind, what are you most scared of? What problems do you need to resolve to succeed? Is this an impulsive risk? Does it endanger or harm anyone else? What's the worst that can happen to you? What can be done to ensure success?*

Sandra and Bill bought a bed and breakfast in the country. Their vision was to create a gathering place for small-business retreats for both individuals and groups. They are both charming people and are known for sponsoring great parties and events. Sandra is a talented decorator and is very capable of remodeling an inn to elegance and comfort. Yet neither one of them enjoys cooking, food shopping, or housekeeping. In order to make their plan viable, their budget had to include funds for a staff to cook and clean daily. Therefore they had to buy an inn that was cheaper than they had originally planned and sell some antiques from their collection. While they are both committed to this inn, they are also committed to defining their own job descriptions to utilize their best talents. They hired excellent cooks and cleaners, giving them free reign to be creative and participate actively in the blossoming of the inn's signature style. Sandra and Bill were smart enough to know that having happy long-term staff people was fundamental to their success. Other people scoffed at their plan, saying that in order to make money you have to be willing to cook and clean yourself. Instead, Sandra and Bill stayed committed to their personal version of this business, focusing on marketing and entertaining, at which they excel.

Personal risks can be equally daunting. Dan wanted to marry Pamela, but she had a difficult eight-year-old daughter. Dan was estranged from his own father and feared he wouldn't be able to be a good parent to Pamela's daughter, especially with her emotional temperament. But he realized that the worst that could happen to him was that he would live without Pamela, and that this was an unacceptable option. They married, he joined a stepfather's support group, and the three of them participated in long-term family therapy.

Many people on their deathbeds regret the things they were too scared to try. Don't be afraid to be afraid. The question is, Are you going to let fear restrict your freedom of choice? Or you are going to analyze the factors you need to incorporate into your risk plan so that it works for you?

Grace and her family loved California. As job transitions loomed on the horizon for both Grace and her husband, they quickly decided to move to where they really wanted to live and enjoy the good weather and lifestyle. This meant leaving both sets of grandparents on the east coast. To guarantee a positive outcome, Grace and her husband bought a place with a guest apartment so that family members could visit for extended periods of time.

Be aware of risks that endanger you, your physical security, health, or all of your financial resources. While there are stories of people successfully investing every single dime into a creative project, a business, or a social movement, too many others lose it all by not facing the reality of their challenges. Be sure that you have a safety net for yourself and that your plan is working well enough to keep going with it. Sometimes there are great lessons to be learned about your own limitations that point to different actions than you had originally anticipated. Don't be too stubborn to ask for help or to dissect the problem. Sometimes scaling down your vision or letting go until you have a stronger foundation of people and monetary resources is a wise move.

So, what kind of preparation and gear do you need to sail around your cliff? Awareness of your strengths and weaknesses and of the possible pitfalls is as essential to a successful sail as a sturdy mast. Prepare yourself, but carefully select your crew of support. Be cautious in forming alliances. It would be wonderful if you could trust everyone, but you can't. Pay attention to every concern that your intuition picks up about a potential partner or contributor. Work on a mini-project first with someone before you dive into a deeper connection. Don't commit your time, energy, or love until the other person has earned your trust. The wrong alliances can put your future into a tailspin for years. Jenna sold her business to a dishonest woman and spent the next few years in litigation. Kirk bought a franchise only to discover a year later that their services were substandard to their biggest competitor. Before you commit, take your time, think it over, and get all the facts. Above all, honor those intuitive messages, even if they are vague and confusing.

Tune into the power of Yes. Your Yeses are Positive Choices. If you are careful about when you say Yes to people, projects, timelines, and tasks, then you will have fewer Subtractions to deal with later. Don't sign up for connections that don't excite you. Be clear about who your true friends and colleagues are.

INQUIRY *With whom do you have mutually supportive relationships? Who is just using you? Who and what do you want as Yeses in your life? Write down all of the people in your life into three categories: (1) true friends, (2) positive acquaintances, and (3) untrustworthy folks and enemies. Then be discriminating about whom you invite to share the ups and downs of your risks.*

Your Yeses are your commitments. The risks that you choose to dance with are your commitments. Your true friends and other positive acquaintances whom you value enough to work with on the dynamics of mutuality are your commitments. Will there be challenges in these relationships? Of course there will be. Determining who supports our risks in life and who doesn't helps us to find the right community of positive risk-takers and distance from negative thinkers. If you are committed to a Positive Choice, you need to locate people who genuinely want you to meet your goals and enjoy helping you achieve your dreams. In turn, you need to be committed to their triumphs as well and available to brainstorm with them when they crave your wisdom and point of view.

Calculated risks are potential catalysts to bring you closer to the life that expresses the true you—the best you.

Chapter 14

E Is for Empathizing

Resolve to be as kind to yourself as your best self is to others. Do you have higher standards for yourself than for other people? Sarah thought that if her next relationship with a man failed she'd never forgive herself. Yet Sarah was always there when her friends broke up with their partners and didn't consider them failures. She needed to learn to be as generous and empathic with herself as she was with others.

Appreciate yourself for the person you are. Are you a good friend, parent, or family member? Are you generous and a good listener or problem solver? Build on your kindness to others by saluting your own goodness. Often the worst abuse of all is self abuse. Perfectionism deprives you of necessary learning-steps along the way to your goal. Do you inflict yourself daily with doubts and criticisms, and focus on your limitations instead of your strengths? Do you torture yourself for not doing things that you're not even ready to do yet? Indecision can be damaging to your self-esteem and create confusion about your true priorities and beliefs.

INQUIRY *Write down all of your self-criticisms for one week and note the patterns. You'll probably be shocked!*

Marty did this exercise and discovered that he was the cause of his own low self-regard. He began his day with unrealistic expectations of what he could accomplish, so he always fell short. As manager of a bakery, he had too much responsibility and incompetent help. The owner was cheap and expected Marty just to get everything done. After working with a coach, Marty realized that in order to be successful, he had to reorganize his entire job and hire motivated employees. A critical inner voice can be helpful at times, like when it reminds us to double-check our math, but Marty's tyrannical inner critic cost him his sense of well-being as well as the confidence to solve his problems.

INQUIRY *Acknowledge yourself by writing down your accomplishments for one week. You'll probably feel better. If not, then it's time to review your priorities.*

Nancy loved her profession as a physical therapist. She recently bought the perfect condo with a greenhouse and a hot tub. But, even with these good things in her life, Nancy realized that her number 1 goal was to make several new long-term friends who were both spiritual and entertaining. She realized, however, that she wasn't reaching out to anyone new. After acknowledging her priorities, she made two Additions to her life. She joined her local garden club and set up three dinner dates with women she liked but didn't know well. At the end of the month, she promised herself a reward—a new orchid plant!

Celebrate your successes, and be gentle with yourself about reaching for new goals. Don't duck what you need to do, but allow yourself to move at a comfortable pace. Bring an empathic energy to yourself as well as to the important people in your life.

How much stress in your life comes from conflicts with dysfunctional others? You have free choice to Subtract certain people from your life, such as idiot bosses or nasty store owners. Your relationships with your family and old friends, however, can be much more complicated, as it's hard to Subtract family members permanently or estrange yourself from old friends. Yet, Subtraction may be the only healthy choice; you need to let go of the past and protect yourself from further disappointments. If you choose to keep some dysfunctional folks in your sphere, you have to accept their limitations and operate within your own safety zone.

Katrina wants to stay connected to her family, even though they disapprove of her lifestyle. So she visits them for short stints and stays with a friend nearby. It takes courage for her to set these kinds of boundaries, but this arrangement is essential for preserving her dignity.

Sometimes a crisis can precipitate a healing experience with difficult people if both parties can meet in the spirit of mutual honesty and allegiance. Until then, bring forth your powers of empathy, forgive them for their short-comings, and release the pain of it.

Fill your life with people you trust and who are capable of enacting relationships based on giving and receiving. Pick a work environment with like-minded others, and link up with folks of similar values. Find other Positive Choices seekers and set up a support group or a buddy system for yourself. Mutually empathic relationships stimulate your sense of abundance. Negative relationships compromise your self-worth, drain your creative urges, and engender emotional turmoil. Is there someone in your life who expects too much from you? By owning your own life plan, you become immune to those projections from others. Build a support community that is reciprocal and loving. Share your wisdom and dreams with others who can learn from you, and in turn foster your growth. Be empathic toward everyone, but reserve the right to choose your entanglements.

Chapter 15

Is for
Synthesizing

You now have the tools to re-create your life with exciting, meaningful, and spirited choices. Each time you Subtract a Serenity Stealer and Add in a Positive Choice, you soar, you grow, you prosper. The bridge of The Same is now only a distant memory. By choosing to take advantage of the power of Positive Choices, you have organically broken from your past. Let's take a moment to synthesize your discoveries.

INQUIRY *Take note of your progress so far. How are you doing with your original five Serenity Stealers and your original five Positive Choices? How many instances of Addition and Subtraction have happened already? Celebrate your completions here. Are you ready to tackle the other items on your lists? Set a timeframe and chart your progress each month. Keep adding new Positive Choices to your list all the time. You want this simple formula to become a habit.*

Be patient. It will take time to turn the tide and harvest all the fruits of the life you fancy. But by using the exchanges of Additions and Subtractions, you will notice a major difference and further engage with the potential of continually elevating your life experience.

INQUIRY *In reviewing the Positive Choices that you have already Added to your life, what are the benefits? Do you feel happier or more serene or more satisfied with your life? By releasing your Serenity Stealers, do you have more of a sense of your own serenity? In what ways? Reinforce your gains by defining why and how these changes enhance your life.*

Keep track of the benefits of your new lifestyle in a running log in the back of your journal. John realized that he was less irritable with his sons, and Marge felt she had tapped into a myriad of new ideas. Before Barbara Adds anything new to her life, she ponders what she needs to Subtract in order to make room. In this fast-paced new frontier of technology, the lives of most people are over-loaded. Unload yours. Start with releasing the junk in your garage or on your computer and progress to letting go of the things in your life that no longer support your beliefs and values, whether it's your workplace or a friend who betrayed you.

As you become more empowered, share this simple secret of Addition and Subtraction with others. If you are a manager, help your employees learn to delegate responsibilities to others so they can advance to more challenging projects. If you are a parent, help your child identify his or her personal style and carefully select activities and relationships that augment his or her goals. Be sure and honor their individuality and encourage their own creative choice-making strategies.

Seek out people who refuse to settle for mediocrity in their lives and lean on each other. This is a new age, and many of the old norms are passé. Questing for security can be a trap. Security is an illusion anyway. Your real security comes from accepting the person you are and investing your time and energy into fortifying your talents and transforming your shortcomings. Don't be afraid to take on the hard challenges. If you want to be a better mother, pour your being into that goal, and make it happen. When you see a side of yourself you don't like, own it, and get the guidance you need to change it. If you want to improve the environment, pick an issue and begin. If you want to mend a relationship, tell the truth. It will be worth it.

The human state is about limitations. None of us lives forever, at least not in this form, and we only have so much energy available in a given day. We have personal limitations in intelligence, skills and aptitudes, learning styles and interests, and emotional development.

These limitations actually create a structure for your life; they highlight the need for total clarity about what you want. Because your resources are limited, capitalizing on your finite energy is all the more vital. You want to get the maximum out of who you are and the time you have. Focus on making room for the goals and dreams that most fulfill you. Keep Adding and Subtracting, enjoy your dances with change, and create new models. Be glad that you chose the bridge of Positive Choices. You've chosen to transform your own life into a jeweled treasure chest.

Acknowledgments

To Leslie Berriman and all the wonderful souls at Conari Press that I have had the pleasure and privilege to work with the past several years: You are an outstanding team. Many thanks for getting this book and *The 12 Secrets of Highly Creative Women: A Portable Mentor* out to a wider audience. We are partners with the same vision, and I am overwhelmed with gratitude that we have made this connection.

To my husband, Rusty Street: Thanks again for your unconditional support and love during all the days of our lives. I am eternally grateful to have you as my life partner. Your support for my creative projects has been unbelievable.

To my family and friends: Once again, I appreciate your words of support and marketing efforts on behalf of both books.

To Liz Murphy, my virtual assistant: You have been an essential part of my success and my sanity this past year. I cannot thank you enough for all that you have done and for affirming that there are angels like you out there.

To the women in my Book Marketing Collaborative: A sincere thank you for your ideas and energy and commitment to our collective success.

To Deborah Knox, Gail Jones, Cheryl Gilman, and Debbie Sosin: A heartfelt thank you for your enthusiasm for this project!

To Marilyn Veltrop: Thank you for just being there each morning, willing to listen to my musings.

Bibliography

Adrienne, Carol. *The Purpose of Your Life.* New York: William Morrow & Co., 1999.

Anderson, Joan. *A Year by the Sea.* New York: Doubleday, 1998.

Breathnach Ban, Sarah. *Simple Abundance: A Daybook of Comfort and Joy.* New York: Warner Books, 1995.
_____. *Something More: Excavating Your Authentic Self.* New York: Warner Books, 1998.

Bry, Adelaide. *Visualization: Directing the Movies of Your Mind to Improve Your Health, Expand Your Mind, and Achieve Your Life Goals.* New York: Barnes & Noble Books, 1978.

Cameron, Julia. *The Artist's Way: A Spiritual Path to Higher Creativity. A Course in Discovering and Recovering Your Creative Self.* New York: Putnam Publishing, 1992.

Capacchione, Lucia, Ph.D., A.T.R. *The Creative Journal: The Art of Finding Yourself.* North Hollywood, CA: Newcastle Publishing Company, 1989.
_____. *Visioning: Ten Steps to Designing the Life of Your Dreams.* New York: Simon & Schuster/Fireside, 1991.

Dolnick, Barrie. *Simple Spells for Success: Ancient Practices for Creating Abundance and Prosperity.* New York: Harmony House, 1996.

Dreamer, Oriah Mountain. *The Invitation.* San Francisco: HarperSanFrancisco, 1999.

Ealy, Dr. C. Diane, and Dr. Kay Lesh. *Our Money Ourselves: Redesigning Your Relationship with Money.* New York: Amacom, 1999.

Fritz, Robert. *The Path of Least Resistance: Learning to Become the Creative Force in Your Own Life.* New York: Fawcett Columbine, 1984.

Gawain, Shakti. *Creating True Prosperity.* Novato, CA: New World Library, 1997.

_____. *Creative Visualization.* New York: Bantam New Age Books, 1982.

_____. *Living in the Light: A Guide to Personal and Planetary Transformation.* Mill Valley, CA: Whatever Publishing, 1986.

_____. *Return to the Garden: A Journey of Discovery.* San Rafael, CA: New World Library, 1989.

Gilman, Cheryl. *Doing Work You Love.* Chicago: Contemporary Books, 1997.

Hagberg, Janet O. *Wrestling with Your Angels: A Spiritual Journey to Great Writing.* Holbrook, MA: Adams Publishing, 1995.

Herman, Emily, and Jennifer Richard Jacobson. *Stones from the Muse.* New York: Fireside, 1997.

Knox, Deborah, and Sandra Butzel. *Life Work Transitions.com: Putting Your Spirit Online.* Boston: Butterworth Heinemann, 2000.

Lloyd, Carol. *Creating a Life Worth Living.* New York: HarperCollins Publishers, 1997.

Louden, Jennifer. *The Comfort Queen's Guide to Life: Create All That You Need with Just What You've Got.* New York: Harmony Books, 2000.

McMeekin, Gail. *Positive Choices: From Stress to Serenity.* Boston: Guided Growth, 1992. (audiocassette)
_____. *The 12 Secrets of Highly Creative Women: A Portable Mentor.* Berkeley, CA: Conari Press, 2000.

Moran, Victoria. *Creating a Charmed Life.* San Francisco: HarperSanFrancisco, 1999.

Murdock, Maureen. *The Heroine's Journey: Woman's Quest for Wholeness.* Boston: Shambhala, 1990.

Orman, Suze. *The Courage to Be Rich.* New York: Riverhead Books, 1999.

Phillips, Jan. *Marry Your Muse: Making a Lasting Commitment to Your Creativity.* Wheaton, IL: Quest Books, 1997.

Ponder, Catherine. *The Dynamic Laws of Prosperity: Forces That Bring Riches to You.* Englewood Cliffs, NJ: Prentice-Hall, 1962.
_____. *Open Your Mind to Prosperity.* Unity Village, MO: Unity Books, 1971.

Richardson, Cheryl. *Life Makeovers.* New York: Broadway Books, 2000.
_____. *Take Time for Your Life.* New York: Broadway Books, 1998.

Robinson, Lynn. *Divine Intuition: Your Guide to Creating a Life You Love.* New York: Dorling Kindersley, 2000.

Rountree, Cathleen. *Coming Into Our Fullness: On Women Turning Forty*. Freedom, CA: The Crossing Press, 1991.
_____. *On Women Turning 50: Celebrating Mid-Life Discoveries*. San Francisco: HarperSanFrancisco, 1993.
_____. *On Women Turning 60: Embracing the Age of Fulfillment*. New York: Three Rivers Press, 1998.

Sheehy, Gail. *New Passages*. New York: Random House, 1995.

Sher, Barbara. *It's Only Too Late If You Don't Start Now: How to Create Your Second Life after Forty*. New York: Delacorte Press, 1998.

Sher, Barbara, and Annie Gottlieb. *Wishcraft: How to Get What You Really Want*. New York: Ballantine Books, 1986.

Sher, Barbara and, Barbara Smith. *I Could Do Anything If I Only Knew What It Was: How to Discover What You Really Want and How to Get It*. New York: Delacorte Press, 1994.

Sinetar, Marsha. *Elegant Choices, Healing Choices*. Mahwah, NJ: Paulist Press, 1988.
_____. *To Build the Life You Want, Create the Work You Love: The Spiritual Dimension of Entrepreneuring*. New York: St. Martin's Press, 1995.

Toms, Justine Willis, and Michael Toms. *True Work: A Sacred Dimension of Earning a Living*. New York: Bell Tower, 1998.

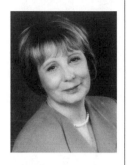

About the Author

Gail McMeekin, M.S.W., is the owner of Creative Success, a career and creativity consulting company. She has more than twenty-five years of experience coaching clients to discover and achieve their personal, professional, and creative goals. Her specialty is empowering people to fulfill their creative potential. As a licensed psychotherapist, career coach, human resources consultant, and writer, Gail has a wealth of knowledge and insight to share with her clients.

Gail has a B.A. from Connecticut College, an M.S.W. from Boston University, and a certificate in Human Resources from Bentley College. She is the author of *The 12 Secrets of Highly Creative Women: A Portable Mentor* (Conari Press, 2000). She has also produced a companion audiocassette workshop to this book called *Positive Choices: From Stress to Serenity,* which has been featured in *The Improper Bostonian* and *Human Resource Executive.* To contact Gail, to order the *Positive Choices* audiocassette and other Creative Success products, or to subscribe to her free e-mail monthly newsletter called *Creative Success,* log onto Gail's Web site at *http://www.creativesuccess.com.*

To Our Readers

Conari Press publishes books on topics ranging from spirituality, personal growth, and relationships to women's issues, parenting, and social issues. Our mission is to publish quality books that will make a difference in people's lives—how we feel about ourselves and how we relate to one another. We value integrity, compassion, and receptivity, both in the books we publish and in the way we do business.

As a member of the community, we sponsor the Random Acts of Kindness™ Foundation, the guiding force behind Random Acts of Kindness™ Week. We donate our damaged books to nonprofit organizations, dedicate a portion of our proceeds from certain books to charitable causes, and continually look for new ways to use natural resources as wisely as possible.

Our readers are our most important resource, and we value your input, suggestions, and ideas about what you would like to see published. Please feel free to contact us, to request our latest book catalog, or to be added to our mailing list.

2550 Ninth Street, Suite 101
Berkeley, California 94710-2551
800-685-9595 • 510-649-7175
fax: 510-649-7190 • e-mail: conari@conari.com
www.conari.com